The New Baby

For Norma

VIKING KESTREL
Viking Penguin Inc., 40 West 23rd Street, New York, New York 10010, U.S.A.
Penguin Books Ltd, Harmondsworth, Middlesex, England
Penguin Books Australia Ltd, Ringwood, Victoria, Australia
Penguin Books Canada Limited, 2801 John Street, Markham, Ontario, Canada L3R 1B4
Penguin Books (N.Z.) Ltd, 182–190 Wairau Road, Auckland 10, New Zealand

First published in 1987 by Viking Penguin Inc.
Published simultaneously in Canada

Manufactured in Singapore by Imago Publishing Ltd.
Set in Garamond #3

1 2 3 4 5 91 90 89 88 87

Library of Congress Cataloging in Publication Data
Young, Ruth, 1946– The new baby.
Summary: When Mom and Dad bring home a new baby, big brother feels apprehensive until he helps Mom care for the newcomer.
[1. Babies—Fiction] 2. Brothers and sisters—Fiction] I. Title. PZ7.Y877Ne 1987 [E]
87-6280 ISBN 0-670-81304-4

The New Baby

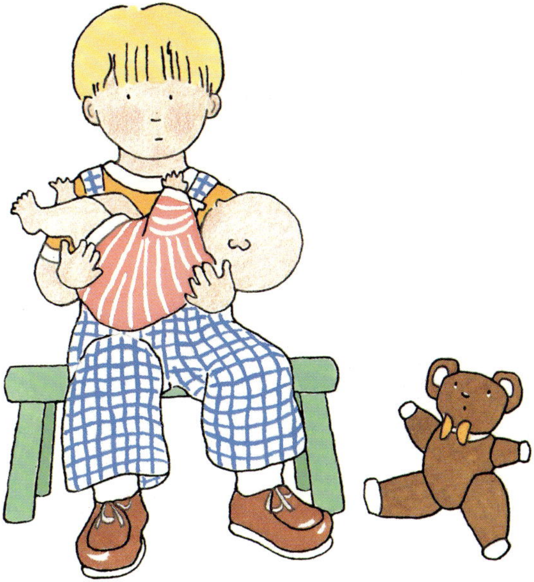

RUTH YOUNG

VIKING KESTREL

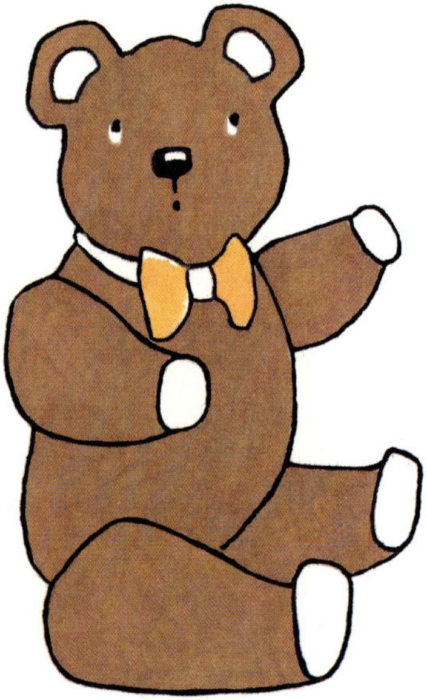

When Mommy and Daddy brought the New Baby home, they brought a new Teddy Bear for me.

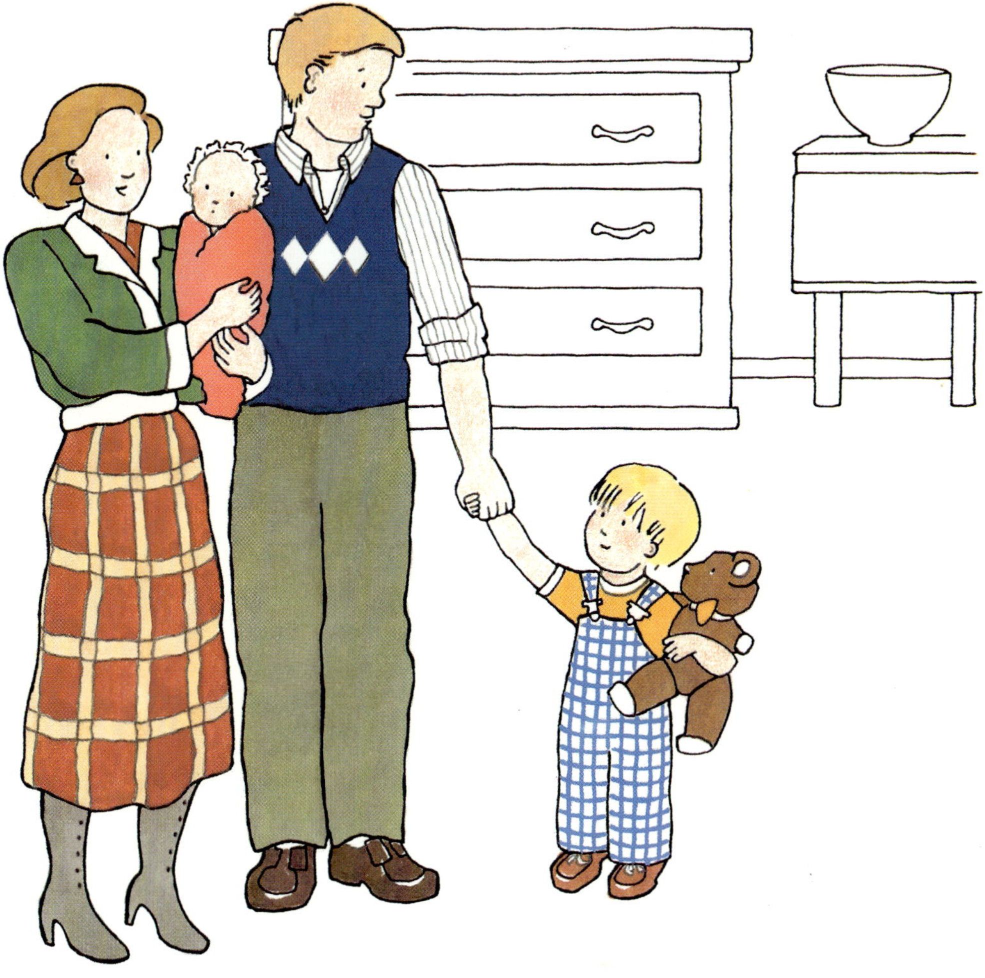

They said I would like the New Baby.

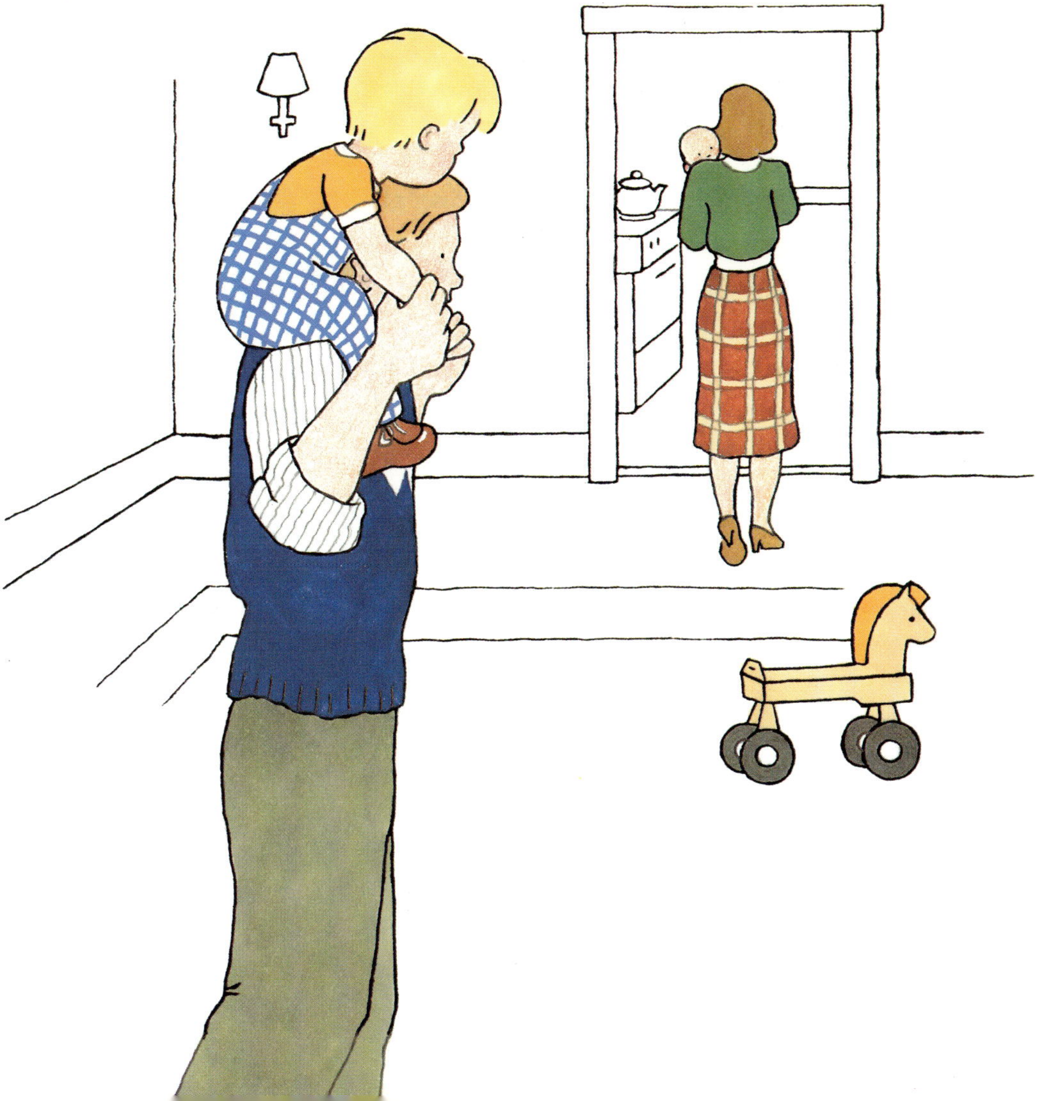

It is very little, with no hair.

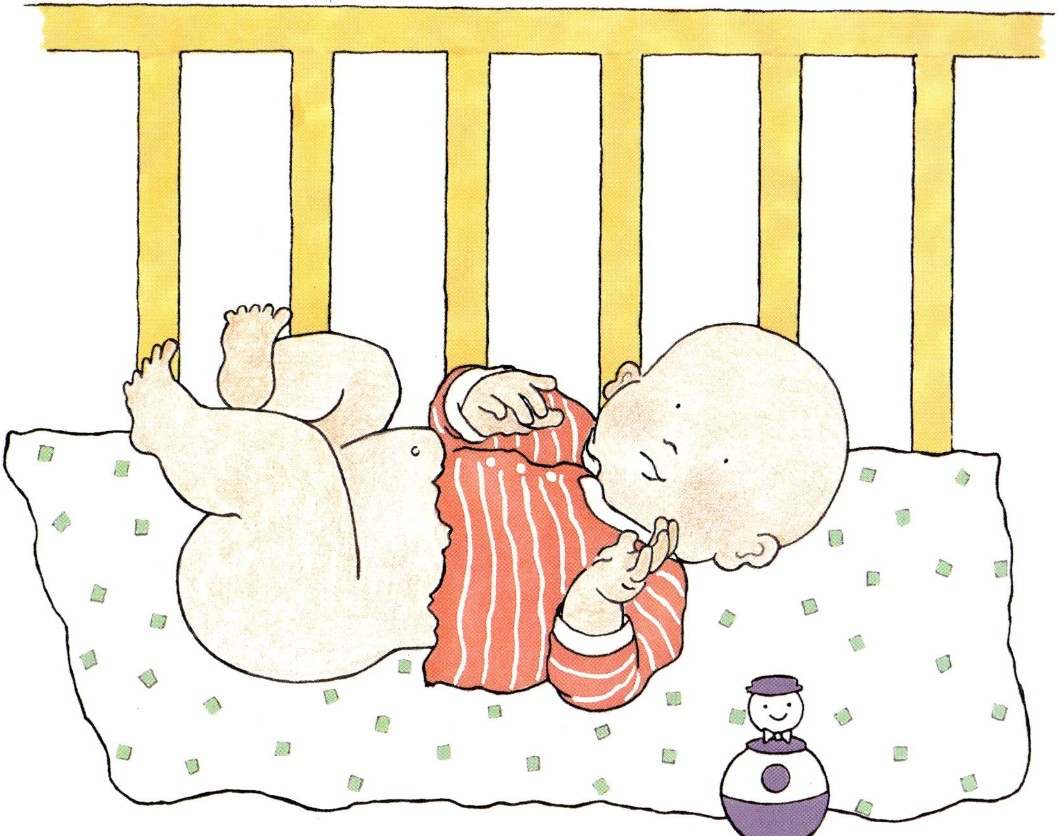

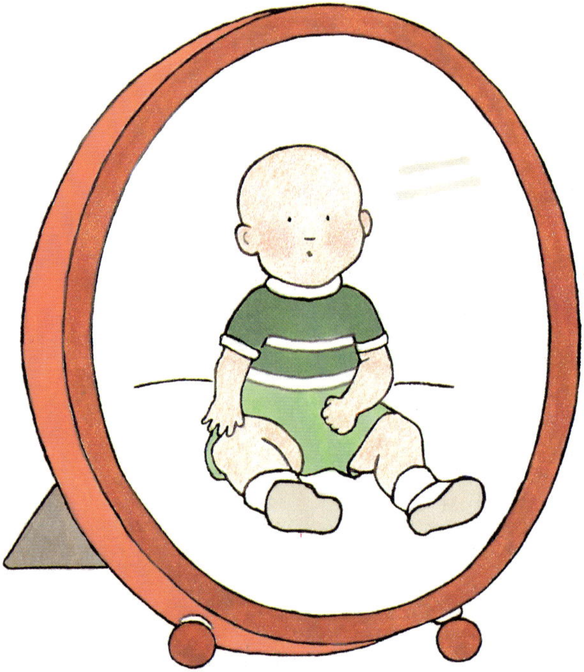

Daddy says I was that way, too.

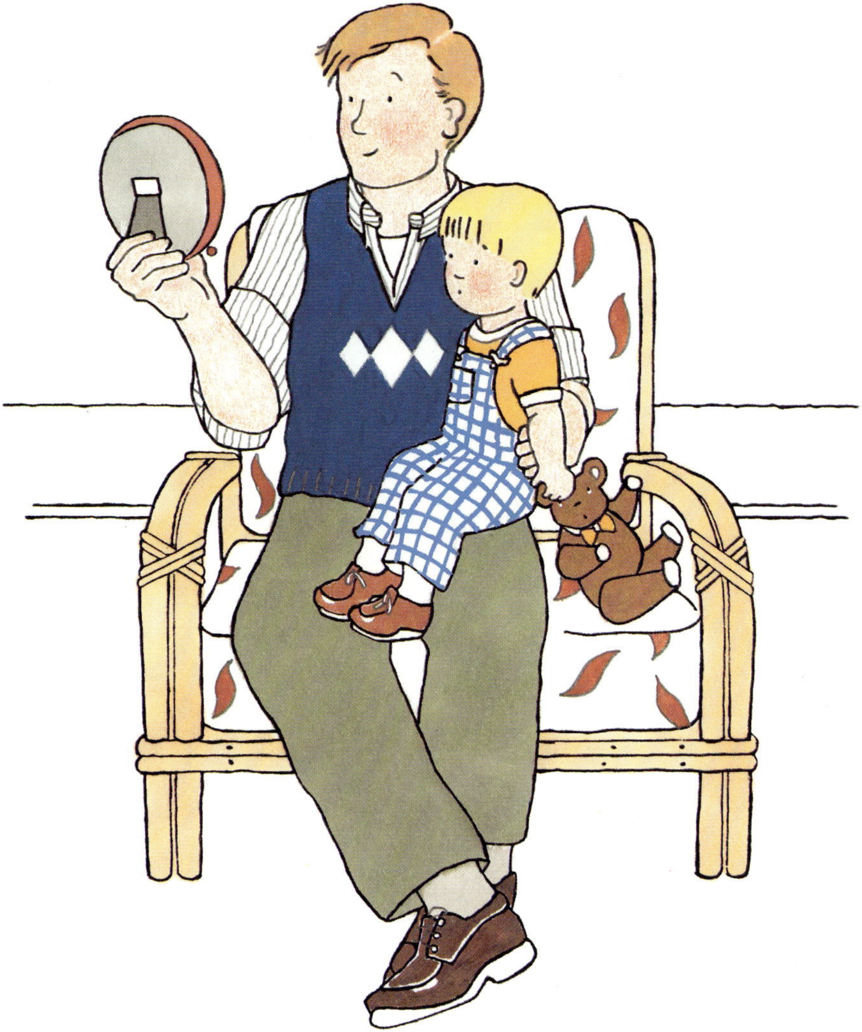

The New Baby can't play very much yet.
But sometimes it laughs if I
make squeaky noises.

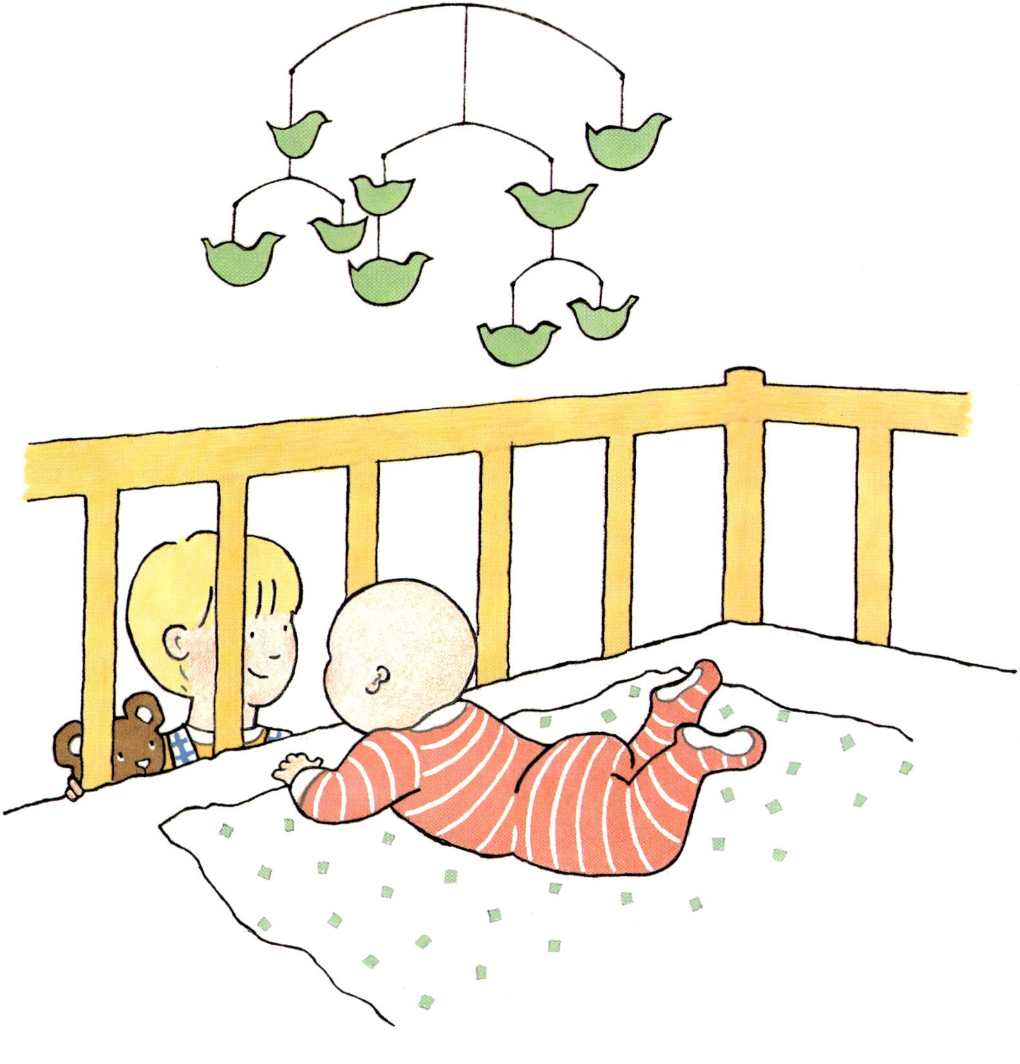

When it has a bath, I help out.

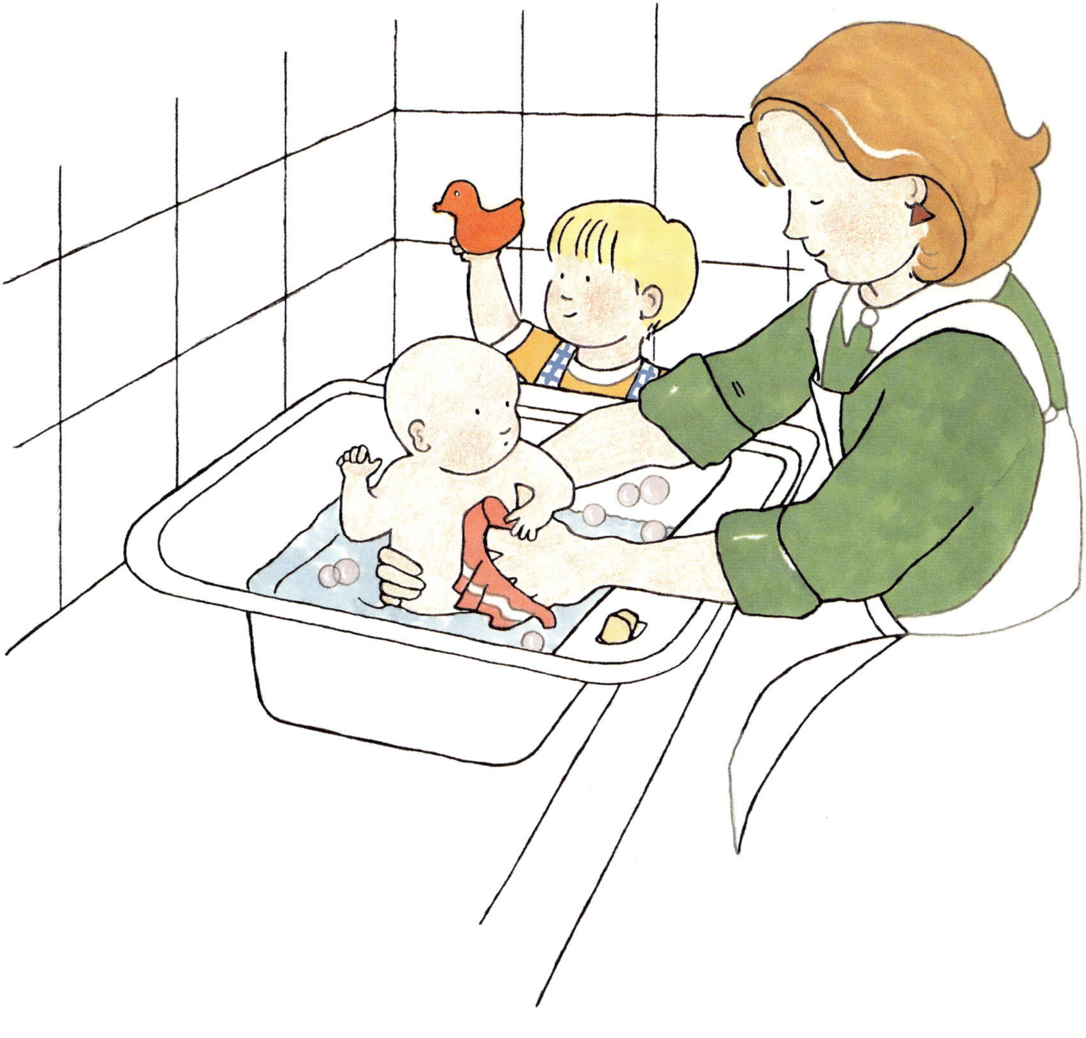

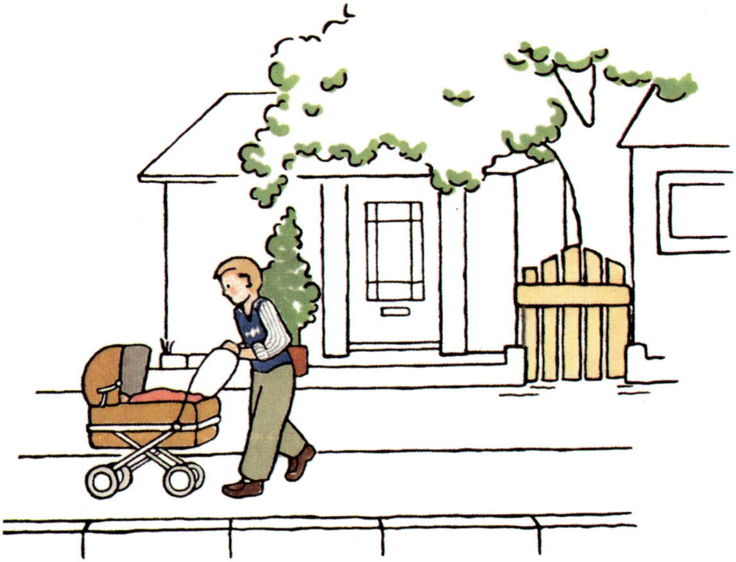

Sometimes I like to be alone with Mommy.
Then Daddy takes the New Baby for a walk.

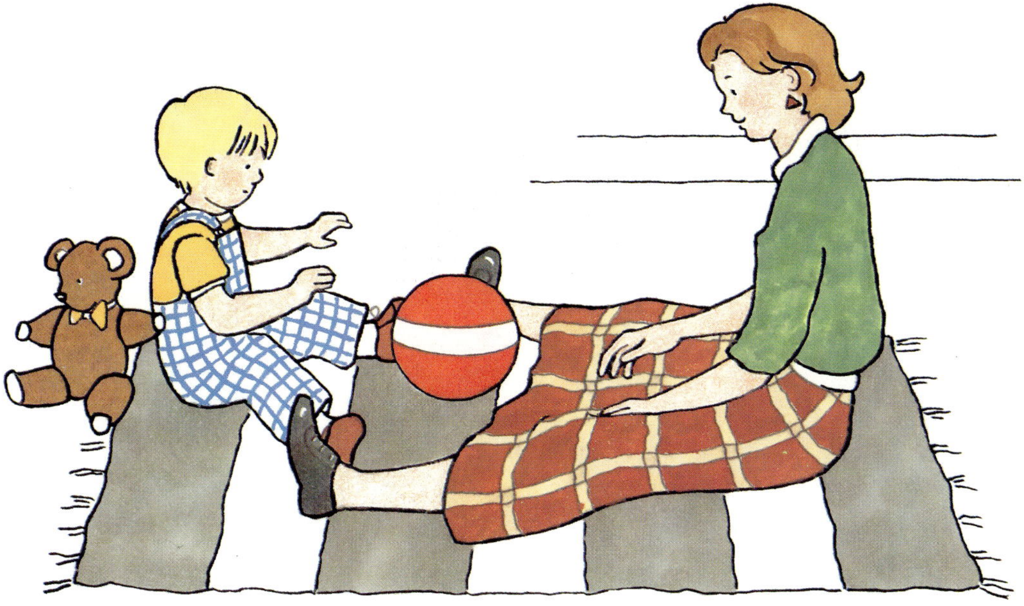

When Mommy and I sing
The Golden Bear Song,
the New Baby always goes to sleep.
Someday when it gets bigger, if I
want to I will teach it how to sing:

"Golden Bear, Golden Bear,
I have seen him Everywhere.
Dancing up the Golden Stair,
Rocking in my Rocking Chair."

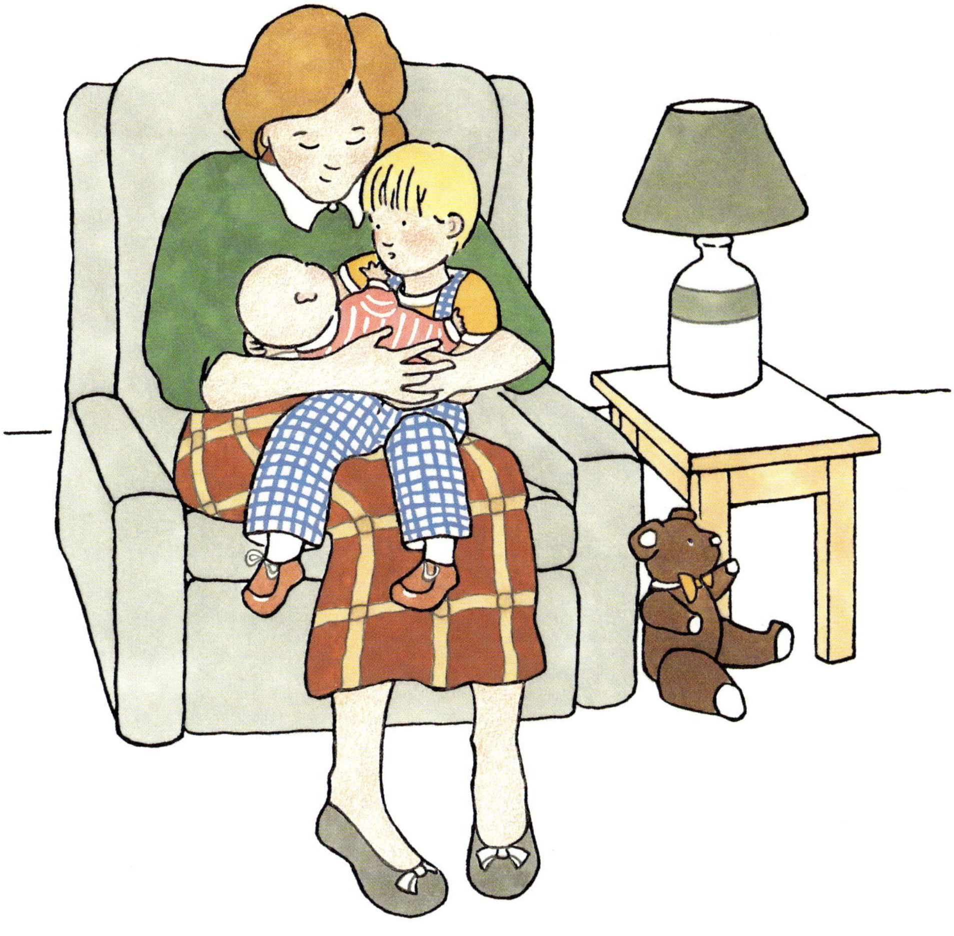

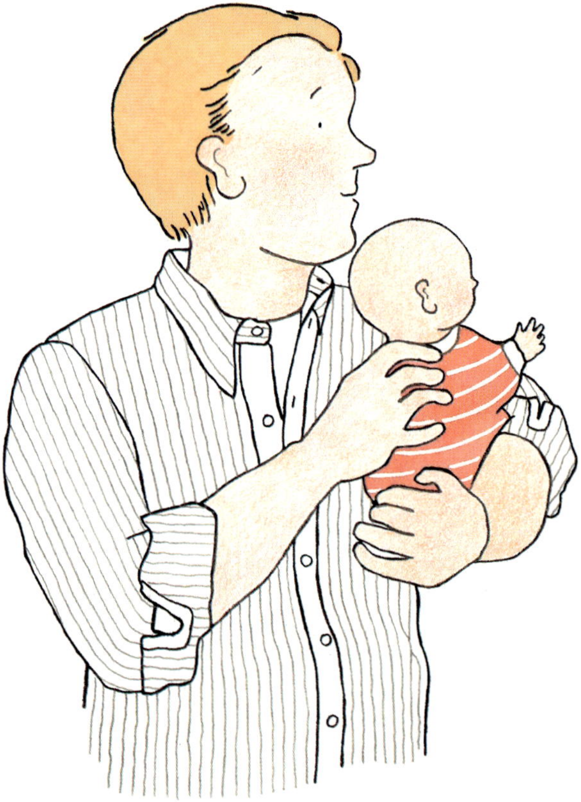

Mommy says the New Baby looks like Daddy.

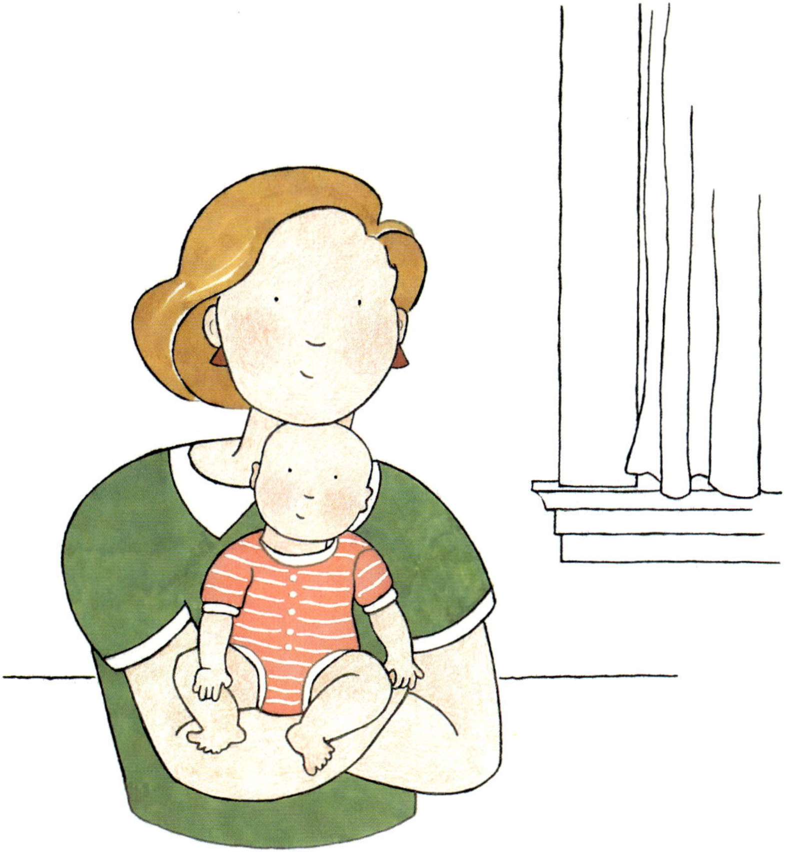

Daddy says it looks like Mommy.

I think it looks like me.

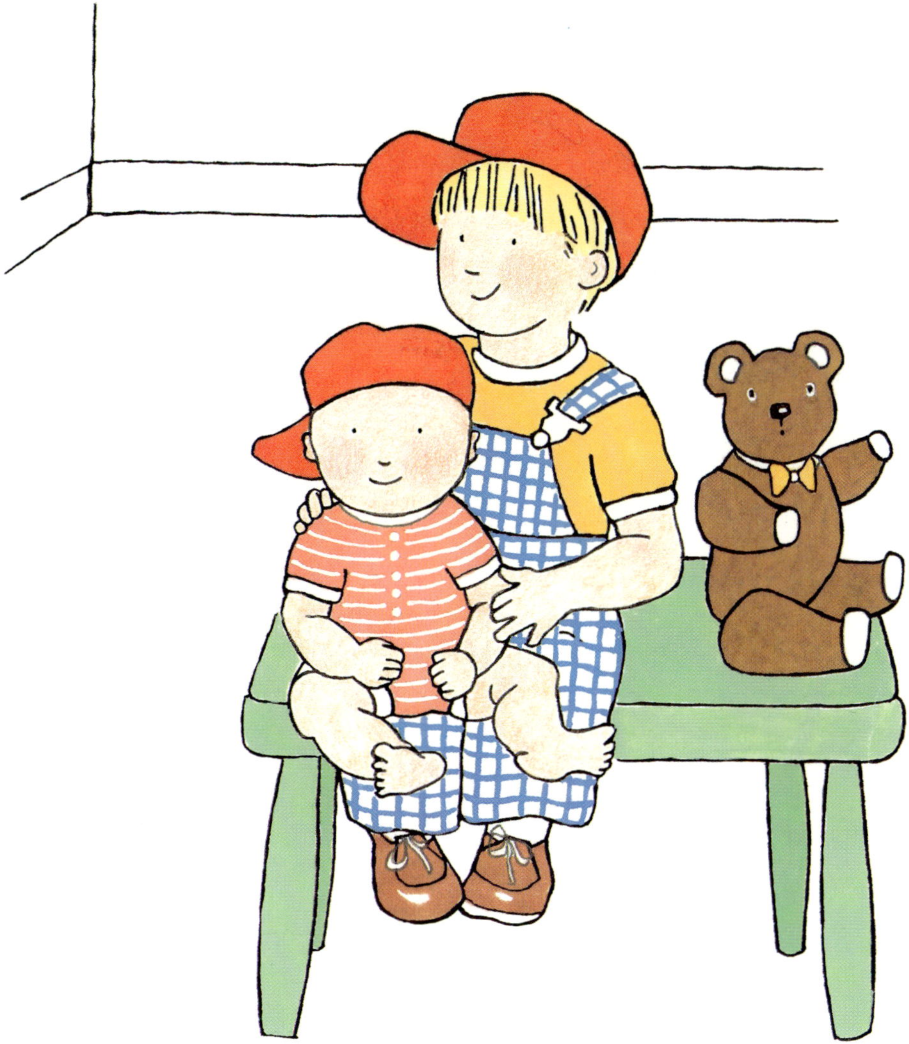